How to Survive Pumping:

Tips to Make Expressing

Breast Milk Easier on You

JENNIFER DAGGETT

ISBN: 1490961399
ISBN-13: 978-1490961392

Contents

A Brief Introduction

I'm a former exclusive pumping mother, so I know how hard it can be. In total, I pumped for 16 months. Sometimes it was okay and sometimes it was so bad I felt I couldn't bear one more second. I thought about quitting more times than I can count and twice I very nearly did. Using the ideas in this book I kept going and achieved my goal.

You too can reach your pumping goal, whatever that is. I wrote this book to try to make it easier for you. Some of the tips in this book worked for me, some for other pumping mothers. Not all of them will work for you, but hopefully enough will to make a real difference in your day-to-day life.

Each chapter in this book deals with a different issue. You can read them in order, or dip in and out, as you choose.

This book assumes that you are already pumping, so doesn't deal with deciding to pump (does anyone?), choosing a pump (other than a few thoughts) or building a milk supply. There are many excellent books on these subjects. I've listed a few you might want to look at in *Chapter 7: Further Reading*.

1. Pumping Takes Up So Much Time

Taking care of a small child is a full-time job. If you're pumping, you pretty much have two of them. Here are some ways to reduce the time you spend pumping.

Your Pump

As a general rule (there are always exceptions – by all means experiment), a double electric pump will take the least time to get the amount of milk you need.

Personally, I hired a hospital-grade pump (a Medela Symphony). Although this is the most expensive option, if I pump for another baby I will not hesitate to do the same again. I knew my pump could take anything I threw at it (I managed to resist the temptation to test this - just) and would get my milk out if anything could.

If you can't afford to hire a pump, or you are only pumping part-time, there are plenty of other options, but I urge you to select your pump with care. A poor quality or worn-out pump will mean more time spent pumping and a much harder time maintaining your supply. If you are having trouble pumping enough milk, try a different (ideally better quality) pump.

If you have private health insurance, it may cover breast pump hire or purchase. In the US, pumping supplies may be tax deductible as medical expenses. Do check, if this will enable you to get a better pump.

A discussion of different pumps is beyond the scope of this book, but you can find reviews of different pumps on sites such as Amazon and Mumsnet. The main pump makers are Medela and Ameda. Lansinoh, Ardo, most of the bottle-makers and some other companies also make pumps.

You may want to have a back-up pump, just in case, and spares of all the parts. Check parts regularly for wear, because a worn part can dramatically reduce your pump's effectiveness.

Pumping Technique

Books on building milk supply will cover this in more detail, but some things that can help you get the milk out faster are:

* Breast massage and compression, before and during pumping;

* Warmth (a hot bath or shower before pumping, a hot water bottle or microwave beanbag over your breasts during);

* A higher pump suction setting (as long as it is comfortable for you);

* Visualising running water or thinking about your baby, to aid let down. If your baby is not with you, photos, something of theirs (e.g. a toy or blanket) that smells like them or a recording of them can help;

* A set pre-pumping routine. This works on the same basis as a bedtime routine, as in it conditions your milk let-down reflex to happen after a series of triggers; and

* Relaxation exercises.

Sterilising

To sterilise your pumping equipment you can put it in a saucepan of water and boil it, you can use a microwave or electric steam steriliser or you can use sterilising fluid in a cold water tank. Some pumps say that their equipment is not suitable for one or more options, usually steaming or boiling, so do check before you buy.

For set up time, sterilising fluid is quickest, then steaming, then boiling. With a cold water tank, you make up new steriliser fluid once a day with cold water (you don't usually need to boil it first) and then just submerge your clean pumping gear. With steaming, you load up the steriliser, add water and either turn it on or stick it in the microwave. For boiling, you obviously need to boil water first.

In terms of sterilising time, steaming is quickest (4-10 minutes depending on the steriliser and/or how powerful your microwave is), then either boiling (usually 10-20 minutes once the water's boiling, but check for your pump) or sterilising fluid (15 minutes to one hour depending on what brand you use).

Some mothers sterilise their pumping equipment before each pumping session and some don't. Since breast milk keeps in the fridge for several days, some mothers wash and sterilise their equipment once a day and then keep it in a sealed container (e.g. a Ziploc bag) in the fridge between sessions. Others wash their pumping gear in hot soapy water (or sling them in the dishwasher – put small parts into a tea strainer or a fine mesh bag to stop them getting lost) between sessions and sterilise them once a day. Many mothers buy several sets of pumping equipment (I've heard of one mother who had fourteen on the go) and sterilise them all at once. This is particularly useful for pumping during the night or at work, since then you don't have to wash up until later. All these options can save you a lot of time.

It's for you to decide what sterilisation routine you are comfortable with, based on your own attitude and the age and health of your baby.

Your Pumping Station

If possible, have a pumping place with everything you need set up there. When my daughter was small, I used to pump in bed. We are lucky enough to have an en suite, which took care of hand-washing, and had a microwave, steriliser, table-top freezer, mini fridge (you can buy all these used to save money) and pump up there. It made things a lot easier, particularly for the middle-of-the-night pumping sessions. If you prefer to pump in a chair or on a sofa, make sure it is comfortable and get yourself a footstool and a table for the pump.

Some other things you might like to have on hand are a drink, a good book, lubricant for the flanges (if you use it) and a hand towel (I used to wrap one around my middle to catch any drips when removing the flanges. If you lean forward when removing them, this will also help). If you make a lot of milk in a single session, have a spare bottle or two within grabbing distance. You don't want to overflow and lose milk.

If you are pumping at work, then privacy is the most important thing. You're going to have trouble letting down if you feel like you're in a goldfish bowl. Ideally, you want a private room with a lockable door. If you work for a very large (or very enlightened) company, there may actually be a mother's room. Failing that, is there a first aid room, a storeroom or a mailroom that you could borrow? If you actually have your own office, can you get blinds?

If you are stuck pumping in a shared workspace, can you get a screen or curtain to go around your desk or cubicle (stick a 'No Entry' sign on while you're pumping)? Can you move to a quieter corner of the office, if there are many people around? At the very least, get yourself a nursing cover and pump with your back to everyone.

Milk Storage

You can buy bottles or bags to store milk. Bottles are more expensive, but in my experience they are much better. It's rare to get a leaking bottle (unless you fill them right to the top and then freeze them – the expansion can split them) and you can usually screw them directly on to your pump so you don't have to pour milk from one container to another. (If your milk goes straight from fridge to baby, you may be able to attach feeding bottles to your pump instead – it depends on the brand(s) of pump and bottles). Bags are handy to have in reserve, though. When defrosting a bag, it's best to put it into a glass in case of leaks.

If you pump at work, keep spare bags or bottles in your desk just in case you forget to bring enough or you make more milk than you expected. Also, don't forget to clearly label anything you put in a communal fridge, or it may end up in somebody's coffee!

If you have a freezer stockpile, here's a tip to cut down on the number of bottles and the amount of freezer space that you need. Since breast milk will keep for several days in the fridge (longer in the main body than in the door) you can keep the milk from one pumping in the fridge and then add the milk from the next one to it. You then put the bottle into the freezer only when it's full (always leave a space at the top to allow for expansion when freezing). Of course, this does mean the milk will be less fresh when it goes into the freezer, so whether it is a good plan depends on how long it will take you to fill a bottle.

Always label your bottles with the date of expression and arrange them by date. That makes it easier to use the oldest stuff first. I used to use plastic bags labelled with marker pen. I also tried using shoeboxes, but found that the bags made better use of the space. If you store your milk in bags, they generally take up the least space if you freeze them flat.

If someone else will be feeding your baby, you may want to store your milk in portions. One good technique is to freeze milk in ice cube trays (also useful for freezing purees when weaning). You can put the cubes into freezer bags once frozen to save space. (If you cover the trays in foil, buy good stuff. I got cheap stuff and I'm still finding bits in the freezer). This way you can just send the relevant number of cubes, to reduce the risk of excess milk being thrown away.

Do explain to any other feeders that it's important to minimise waste. Some people who are not familiar with breastfeeding think that your milk supply is limitless and on tap. It's better to have a chat beforehand than to serve a lengthy jail term for killing them when they tip your precious milk down the drain!

How Often Do You Need To Pump?

For at least six weeks (some experts recommend three months), concentrate on building up your supply and pump as often as you can (at least eight times a day, no more than four hours between sessions).

After your supply is well established, you can experiment. Some mothers can drop a number of sessions without a drop in supply (it's best to do this gradually to reduce the risk of blocked ducts and mastitis). I found I could maintain my supply on six sessions, but some lucky mothers can manage on three or even less. Some even pump more milk when they pump less often, although they are definitely the exception. Some need longer sessions when they pump less often and some don't – the important thing is to empty the breast.

The best way to work out what you need to do is to keep a note of when you pump, how long you pump for and how much you make, as well as how much your baby eats and how much you throw away. Over a few weeks/months, you can work out the minimum you can get away with to keep up with your baby.

Although the amount they need will increase (and you will see temporary increases during growth spurts), because breast milk is used so efficiently by your baby's body they will probably never need as much as they would with formula. Of course, this depends on your baby so it's best to produce a little more than they need if you can.

Milk Leftovers

When my daughter was tiny, I threw away any breast milk left in the bottle after she had fed. It wasn't until I was tracking how much I was producing and feeding her (as I mentioned above) that I realised just how much precious milk I was throwing away. I looked into it and it turns out that most people agree that you can keep leftover breast milk for the next feeding. This is because the active ingredients in breast milk slow the growth of bacteria compared to in formula milk.

Not everyone agrees with this and you may not feel comfortable with it, especially if your baby is very young or ill. However, keeping leftovers can dramatically reduce the amount of milk you throw away and so the amount you have to pump. I've never seen any negative effect on my daughter from doing it.

As I mentioned in *Milk Storage* above, if you will be handing milk over to someone else then take a minute to explain your leftover policy to them.

2. I Feel So Tied Down

When you have a million things to do, having to sit down and pump multiple times a day is the last thing you need. Here are some ideas to get more freedom.

Go Hands-Free

Hands-free pumping is essential if you're going to pump for any length of time (after several weeks of pumping eight times a day I'd developed carpal tunnel syndrome from holding the flanges in place) and it's easy to achieve.

The first option is to buy a special hands-free pumping bra. There are quite a few out there. They tend to be a bit pricy, so shop around. Do check before you buy if they can accommodate breast massage/compression, because this can really help in getting milk out faster.

The second option is to get a cheap stretchy sports top (or any tight, stretchy bra you don't mind sacrificing) and cut a couple of holes in it to put the flanges through. (NB I've seen some mothers say that this doesn't work if you have large breasts. Well, I was wearing a 38H nursing bra – and it was still too small – and I got on just fine, so try it and see). The holes will stretch over time unless you sew around the edges, but mine still saw out a year. Get two so you can have one in the wash. I found they got less stretchy with wear, but bounced back when washed.

The third option, which I haven't tried but apparently works, requires only two elastic ponytail bands for each side, so is even cheaper. For more information see Kelly Mom's explanation (see *Chapter 7: Further Reading*), which has step-by-step instructions and pictures.

Pumping bras generally fit over your nursing bra. You will need to take your top off to put it on, so avoid wearing anything with fiddly fastenings. In winter, a cardigan or zip-up fleece is useful. To keep your middle warm, you can use a blanket, a towel (also useful for catching drips) or a leftover bump warmer from your pregnancy.

Go Plug-Free

Most electric pumps are capable of running on batteries, which means you don't need to stay within range of a plug socket. Some are actually designed to be carried around with you, such as the Medela Pump in Style. Others can be adapted for this by getting a small backpack (some pump makers also sell these, but a cheap one from the supermarket will probably work just fine).

Two things to check if you're doing this: one, that the pump tubes are long enough to reach from breast to backpack and two, the weight of your pump. Some of them are rather heavy to be carrying around for any length of time, particularly hospital-grade ones. If your budget will stretch to it, you might want to consider a second pump for carrying around.

If you're going to be bending down, check your pumping equipment. The set I had for my Medela Symphony had holes at the back so if I leant forward the milk would leak out (which is a major design flaw). Strangely enough, it didn't occur to me until writing this book that I could have covered the holes up with tape. If you have this pump, try it and let me know if it works.

Go Mobile

Some pumps have accessories that allow you to plug them into car batteries. These will cost extra (and are not cheap in my experience), but will allow you to get out on the road with your pump. Some mothers actually pump while driving. If you're parked, just remember to keep the engine running to avoid a flat battery.

For sterilisation, a tub with a clip-on lid will make a good portable cold water tank. You can also buy disposable microwave bags (check in advance if there is a microwave you can use) and disposable cold water steriliser bags (which are designed to hang off something stationary so are not ideal for cars, but okay for hotel rooms). Check if the sterilising fluid needs rinsing off before use, in which case you'll also need some cooled boiled water.

For milk storage, a cooler bag/box and a freezer block or similar are required. You may want a nursing cover if you're going to be driving or parked somewhere public. Some places do have somewhere you can pump. If you are going somewhere specific, it's worth asking before you go if they have a mother's room or a first-aid room or similar that you can use. The worst they can say is no.

It does take a while to set up, but at least it means a day trip is possible (if you can actually find the energy).

3. Pumping Hurts

Adjust Your Pump Settings

The first thing to try is to turn down your pump suction to what is comfortable for you. The recommended setting is usually the strongest *comfortable* suction. You may find that you can turn it up after a minute or two, but some mothers actually find they extract more milk at a lower setting, probably because they're more relaxed.

With some pumps, you can buy different-sized or soft-fit flanges. Quite honestly they didn't seem to make any difference to me, but they do to some mothers.

Heal Damaged Nipples

If your nipples are damaged, breast milk itself has healing properties so don't dry your breasts after pumping (unless you have thrush, in which case they need to be kept as dry as possible).

If you are buying a nipple cream, look for one you don't have to remove before breastfeeding such as pure lanolin. You can also rub nipple cream, breast milk (if you can spare any) or olive oil inside the flanges to reduce friction.

I found bathing my nipples in salt water helped them heal faster. A plastic eggcup works quite well as a nipple bath, although you may not want to use it for eggs again.

You can buy breast shells, which you put inside your bra to stop your sore nipples rubbing on your clothes. Read the small print, as the ones I had said you weren't supposed to wear them for more than an hour at a time, which wasn't terribly helpful. Go topless if you can and let your nipples air.

Nipple Infections

If your nipples haven't healed after a few days, or they seem to improve and then get worse again, you may have a nipple infection. You will need to see your doctor for some medicated cream.

Nipple infections can be either thrush or bacterial infections. It's very important to get your doctor to do a swab to confirm which, and not just because they require different cream. If you have thrush, you may not want to keep the milk you pump from that breast *for later use* because of the risk of passing thrush on to your baby (you can feed it to your baby while you are being treated). Do your own research before you decide, since obviously throwing away milk is not to be done lightly. To start you off, read the information at Kelly Mom and La Leche League (see *Chapter 7: Further Reading*).

Mastitis

Mastitis is the bane of every breastfeeding and pumping mother. Usually you will feel like you have the flu (exhaustion, aches and pains, general feelings of crappiness). The infected breast will generally feel hard, hot and painful and the skin will look red (though if you catch it early enough you may be able to avoid the worst of this).

Mastitis can be infectious (in which case you need antibiotics to clear it up) or non-infectious (in which case you don't). Unfortunately, the only way to be sure what kind you have is to wait and see if it gets better on its own. Personally, I just went and got the antibiotics as soon as I figured out what I had, because it was quicker, but you are welcome to wait it out if you prefer. Antibiotics in your milk may give your baby a mild stomach upset, although they didn't seem to bother mine at all.

To treat, keep your breast as empty as possible (i.e. pump as often as you can, every two hours if possible, and massage it as best you can through the pain). Get as much rest as you can (if at all possible, find a babysitter and stay in bed all day). Drink lots of fluids, warm your breasts (bath, shower, hot water bottle or microwave beanbag), avoid tight clothes and go braless if you can. Paracetamol and ibuprofen (but not aspirin) are generally considered safe while breastfeeding.

4. Pumping Makes Me Feel Bad

As if the physical pain wasn't enough, pumping mothers often have to deal with emotional pain as well. Guilt is the most common and most pumping mothers will experience it sometimes. You may feel that pumping takes up time and attention that should go to your baby, your partner, your home, your work, your other children, etc. etc. etc. I don't know any way to deal with this other than to accept that guilt is an inevitable part of being a mother. You are doing something valuable by pumping; you are not wasting time. If it were a waste of time, no one would do it.

Breastfeeding Conditions

For some mothers, however, the negative feelings go beyond guilt. The physical act of pumping actually provokes negative emotions in them. I'm talking here about Breastfeeding Aversion (BA), Dysphoric Milk Ejection Reflex (D-MER) and Sad Nipple Syndrome (SNS).

Breastfeeding Aversion

Some mothers who are pumping while they are pregnant, or are feeding an older child (particularly if they are feeding a baby at the same time), find they dread it. Mothers can feel repulsed, as if their skin is crawling or they are doing something wrong. This generally lasts for the whole session, but may be worse at some times than others.

Dysphoric Milk Ejection Reflex (D-MER)

If you suffer from D-MER, you experience negative emotions when your milk lets down. The feelings last no more than a couple of minutes after let down. D-MER is believed to be caused by a mother's dopamine levels dropping.

Sad Nipple Syndrome (SNS)

Sad Nipple Syndrome is sometimes confused with D-MER, but if you suffer from SNS then you experience negative emotions during the whole time you are pumping, because the trigger is nipple stimulation, not milk let down. You probably dislike any kind of nipple stimulation, including breastfeeding and sexual touching. Some women even find the sensation of clothing grazing their nipples uncomfortable. There is insufficient information available to say what causes SNS.

Living With These Conditions

If you suffer from any of these conditions, pumping is going to be even harder for you than it is for most women. You will need to be very committed/determined/stubborn and find strength to endure the bad feelings. It is possible, however. I suffer from SNS and I still managed to achieve my pumping goal. There are plenty of other women (and some men) out there who feel like this. You are not alone.

Here are some ideas that might help you:

Distraction

Distraction is your best tool in pumping with BA, D-MER or SNS. Go hands-free at least (see *Chapter 2: I Feel So Tied Down*) and go on your laptop, read, watch TV, have conversations, play with your baby or listen to music. Save your favourite shows, books or websites for pumping time. You may need to focus on what you are doing to achieve let down, but for the rest of the time you need to be thinking of anything but if you're going to get through it.

Education & Support

I found it helpful to think of these feelings as 'fake', generated by a medical condition outside my control, rather than actually being about my baby, my life or myself. Suffering from any of these conditions does not mean that you don't love your baby, that you aren't a good mother or even that you're suffering from post-natal depression (although some unlucky people suffer from PND as well).

Making contact with other mothers going through the same thing is helpful. A search/post on an active breastfeeding or pumping forum (see *Chapter 6: Motivation and Support*) should achieve this.

Talking Therapies

For sufferers of BA and SNS (with D-MER the short time the feelings continue for make it less suitable), it may be worth talking to your doctor about cognitive behavioural therapy, which is a technique that helps you keep control of negative thoughts and stop them spiralling out of control.

Some sufferers of BA or SNS (by no means all) have suffered sexual abuse or other bad experiences. There is no evidence that I know of to say if there is a link, but if you know that this has happened to you it may be worth trying psychotherapy.

Natural Therapies

There is precious little information for BA and SNS, but there is a fair bit for D-MER that may also help for these conditions. I discovered D-MER late in my pumping life, so haven't tried any of these myself, but if I pump for another baby believe me I'll be trying everything.

Some things that have been found to have a positive effect on D-MER are Rhodiola (a herb also known as Roseroot or Golden Root), placenta encapsulation, B vitamins, acupuncture, drinking more water, getting more sleep (easier said than done), exercise, pumping alone and getting a bit of me-time.

Some things that tend to make D-MER worse are excessive caffeine (though a small amount can actually help), orgasm and stress.

D-MER.org has more information, plus various other natural treatments you can try including diet changes, herbs and alternative therapies (see *Chapter 7: Further Reading*).

Medication

In severe cases of D-MER, medication that raises a mother's dopamine levels can help. At the time of writing, the front-runner is Bupropion. By contrast, some medication that blocks dopamine receptors may make it worse. If you are taking medication, check with your doctor that it doesn't have this effect. D-MER.org has more information about this (see *Chapter 7: Further Reading*).

Taking medication obviously raises concerns about it getting into your milk. Some medication is established as being unsafe for breastfeeding mothers, but for most there is no clear guidance. If you are considering medication talk to your doctor, research and decide whether the benefits outweigh the risks.

The InfantRisk Center advises on medication use during pregnancy and breastfeeding and has published *Medications and Mothers' Milk*, the details of which are in *Chapter 7: Further Reading*. There are various drug databases online, but be warned that in my experience they often contradict each other.

Weaning

Whatever you do, if you suffer from BA, D-MER or SNS you are going to suffer emotional pain while pumping for your baby. Only you can decide if it's worth doing and, if so, for how long. If pumping is doing significant damage to your mental health or your relationship with your baby, stopping pumping may be the best thing to do. Breast milk benefits babies, but miserable, depressed, angry or resentful mothers do not.

If you are at this point, first consider reducing the amount you pump and combining breast and formula feeding. Your baby will still benefit from the breast milk, but the burden on you will be reduced. You may find that this is enough to enable you to cope.

If it isn't and you do decide to stop, make peace with that decision and congratulate yourself for keeping going as long as you have. You had a major disadvantage in tackling an already difficult task and you have done a wonderful job.

5. My Baby Hates Me Pumping

Children really can be ungrateful little sods sometimes, can't they? Here you are busting a gut to give them the best start in life and all they do is cry, pull on your tubes and try to upset the pump. Pumping is hard enough anyway, but it's ten times worse when you're dealing with the added stress of a complaining baby.

Here are some things you can try:

Pump While Your Baby is Sleeping

I know there are a million things you want/need to do when they're asleep, but if you have a pump-hater this is by far the easiest approach. Obviously, the more often your baby naps the more effective this is. Going hands-free and plug-free (see *Chapter 2: I Feel So Tied Down*) will let you make best use of the time.

Pump While Your Baby is Eating

When my daughter was small, I used to feed and pump in bed. I would sit cross-legged on the bed, put her in my lap, get hooked up to the pump and then bottle-feed her at the same time (alternatively you can prop your baby up on some pillows or in a bouncy chair). She would generally behave while she was eating, although once she got a bit older she started yanking on the tubes when she'd finished. Then I put her down beside me with some toys while I finished pumping. This was okay until she was old enough to start trying to crawl off the bed. You keep adapting.

If your baby is on solids, pump while they're in the highchair. Not only will they be distracted by food, but they also can't get to the pump to interfere.

Save Their Favourite Toys/Activities for Pumping Time

If there is something your baby gets absorbed in for a long while, whether it's a toy, a TV show or watching their clothes spin dry, save it for pumping time. For younger babies, a swing or bouncy chair may keep them happy.

Pay Them Focused Attention Before Pumping

If you think your baby's problem with the pump is that it takes your attention away from them, try spending 15-20 minutes before pumping solely focused on them. Turn off the TV, ignore the computer and your phone and do whatever they like best. You may want to give it five minutes before starting pumping, so they don't associate the pump with the end of this time.

If you go hands-free and plug-free, you can try doing this at the same time as pumping. See *Chapter 2: I Feel So Tied Down* for more information.

Reward/Bribe Them

For a child old enough to understand, you can offer a reward for good behaviour (or, even better, entertaining a younger sibling) while you are pumping. You may need quite a list of ideas to make this work.

Take Advantage of Visitors

If someone comes to visit, pump while they keep your baby busy. You can go into another room (don't worry, I'm not suggesting you get your boobs out in front of your in-laws).

If you have a partner and they are home, they should be entertaining the baby while you pump. Tell them I said so.

Change the Pump Noise

Occasionally a sensitive baby may dislike, or be scared of, the noise your pump makes. Try sticking a blanket or a pillow over the pump to muffle the noise.

There is a fair bit of variation between pumps, so if you've tried everything else it may be worth getting a different one. Read reviews on Amazon and the like (see *Chapter 1: Pumping Takes Up So Much Time*) and see what users say about noise levels. You could try borrowing one or buying a used one to test if it makes any difference before investing in a new one.

6. Motivation and Support

Here are some approaches to help you get through the worst of days.

Why Are You Pumping?

Make a list of the reasons why you want to keep pumping. Tape it to the fridge, or wherever you'll see it often.

You don't have to stick to baby-benefits either. 'It'll help me lose weight' and 'Everyone keeps telling me how I'm superwoman for doing it' are perfectly acceptable reasons. If it motivates you, stick it down. If you don't want anyone else to see it, write it in code. This is all for you; it makes no difference to your baby why you're doing it.

How Long Are You Pumping For?

How long do you want your baby to have your milk for? There's no right answer. Set your goal and then COMMIT TO IT. What got me through the worst days was knowing how bad I would feel if I didn't do what I set out to do. If you are goal-orientated, this may just make the difference.

Set a Waiting Period

An alternative, if you're more of a day-by-day type of person or your goal just feels like too much right now, is to set a waiting period (e.g. a week) between when you decide you want to quit and when you are allowed to do it. Hopefully, by the time the waiting period is over things won't seem quite so bad.

Distraction

See *Chapter 4: Pumping Makes Me Feel Bad.*

Your goal is just to get through each pumping session. Do ANYTHING that helps you (so long as it won't harm you or your baby). Just get through it. Don't worry about the next one until you have to.

Set a Reward

Think up something you really want and promise to get/do it when you reach your pumping goal (NB do discuss it with your partner – if you have one – if it will require a lot of time/money). You can also have smaller rewards for completing each month/week/day/session along the way if you like.

Ask Someone for Support

Only call friends and family if you know they'll encourage you to carry on. Many people will tell you not to feel guilty about quitting and how well you've done to get this far. When you do decide to stop, they'll be great to have around. Right now, not so much.

There may be a breastfeeding group in your local area, although there is no guarantee that any of the mothers there will be pumping. If your baby was premature, there may be a local premature baby group you can join where you should find other mothers who pump or have done (ask at the hospital).

Unfortunately, I haven't found any dedicated pumping help lines (if you find one, please let me know), but hopefully the breastfeeding ones will be able to offer encouragement.

UK
National Breastfeeding Helpline 0300 100 0212
Breastfeeding Network Supporterline 0300 100 0210
NCT Breastfeeding Helpline 0300 330 0771
La Leche League 0845 120 2918
Association of Breastfeeding Mothers 0844 412 2949

US
National Breastfeeding Helpline 800-994-9662 (TDD 888-220-5446)
La Leche League USA 1-877-4-LALECHE (1-877-452-5324)

Helplines for other countries are available at Kelly Mom (see *Chapter 7: Further Reading*).

If you find it hard to ask for help, you are not alone. I have the same problem and am still not that good at it, but this is a skill you need to develop as a mother, pumping or otherwise. Keep trying to get better at it.

Go Online for Support

You may well be the only pumping mother you know, but you are by no means the only one out there. The Internet is the easiest way to connect with others in your position. Every pumping mother has thoughts about quitting. Many on a daily basis, some on an hourly. Go to a message board and ask for advice and encouragement.

Try:

iVillage(US) http://www.ivillage.com/forums/
Exclusively Pumping or Working and Pumping

BabyCenter (US) http://community.babycenter.com/
Pumping Moms

BabyCentre (UK) http://community.babycentre.co.uk/
Pumping Mummies

7. Further Reading

Websites

Exclusively Pumping
http://www.exclusivelypumping.com/
This site is linked to the book *Exclusively Pumping Breast Milk* listed below.

Mother-2-Mother
http://www.mother-2-mother.com/ExclusivePumping.htm

Kelly Mom
http://kellymom.com/

La Leche League International
http://www.llli.org/

The Breastfeeding Network
http://www.breastfeedingnetwork.org.uk/

D-MER.org
http://d-mer.org/

InfantRisk Center
http://www.infantrisk.com/
Information on medication use during pregnancy and breastfeeding. This site is linked to the book *Medications and Mothers' Milk* listed below.

Express Yourself Mums (UK)
http://www.expressyourselfmums.co.uk/
A one-stop shop for pumping gear, including hospital-grade pump hire.

BreastPumps.com (US)
https://www.breastpumps.com/
A pumping gear shop for US mothers.

Sante Mama (US)
http://www.santemama.com/breast-pump-rental/

Hospital-grade breast pump rental.

NB These are not the only places where you can buy/hire pumping gear. They may not be the cheapest or the best. I'm not endorsing them, just giving you a place to start. I am not affiliated with any of them.

Books

The Womanly Art of Breastfeeding by La Leche League International
Aimed at breastfeeding mothers, but has some valuable advice on pumping. This is the book I followed and it worked for me.

The Breastfeeding Mother's Guide to Making More Milk by Diana West and Lisa Marasco
If you're having trouble pumping the amount your baby needs, read this book.

Exclusively Pumping Breast Milk: A Guide to Providing Expressed Breast Milk for Your Baby by Stephanie Casemore
I haven't read this book myself, but the reviews are very good. This book is linked to the Exclusively Pumping website listed above.

Medications and Mothers' Milk 2012 by Thomas W. Hale PhD
Reference book on which medications are safe to use during breastfeeding. This book is linked to the InfantRisk Center website listed above.

NB These are not the only books available. By all means look in your preferred book shop for others.

Author Notes

Thank you for reading this book. I hope you've found it useful and that it will make your pumping life easier.

I would be very grateful if you would leave a quick review on Amazon. Reviews basically determine whether anyone buys this book, so if it has helped you please let others know that it's worth reading.

If you have a great tip that isn't included here, email me at jennifer.daggett1@gmail.com and let me know. If I get enough, I'll do a second edition.

Keep going. You can do it. And the day will come when you can put the pump away (or smash it to pieces if you so choose) and be proud that you did what you set out to do.

Jennifer

About the Author

Jennifer Daggett was thrown into exclusive pumping when her daughter arrived three months early. She managed to push on for sixteen months, through two lots of mastitis, one nipple infection and a permanent case of sad nipple syndrome, mostly due to a stubborn refusal to be beaten. She thinks any mother who pumps for more than a week should get a medal.

She lives with her husband and daughter (who is doing just fine) in North Yorkshire, England.

www.ingramcontent.com/pod-product-compliance
Lightning Source LLC
Chambersburg PA
CBHW052027280526
45793CB00005B/1154